FENUGREEK

MARIAN KIM

ISBN: 1508599017

ISBN-13: 978-1508599012

CONTENTS

1

PROPERTIES

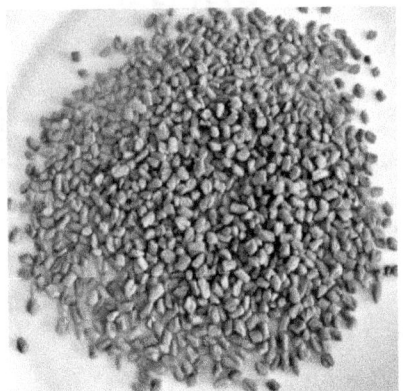

Scientific name: Trigonella foenum-graecum

Other names: Greek hay, Greek clover, bird's foot, fenigreek

Nutrients: Protein, vitamins B3 (niacin) and C. It also contains minerals like potassium. Fenugreek also contains diosgenin which has similar properties to estrogen.

Properties

Antioxidant properties which protect the cells from the free radical damage that causes premature aging and degenerative diseases.

Estrogen-like properties

*, *, *, *, *

2

USES

Diabetes treatment

Fenugreek when taken with meals lowers blood sugar levels in persons with type 1 and 2 diabetes. A study published in the European Journal of Clinical Nutrition found that patients with type 1 diabetes who took 50 grams of fenugreek seed powder twice a day had lower blood glucose levels than those who did not.

High cholesterol treatment

Fenugreek seeds lower the levels of high total cholesterol and low density lipoprotein (LDL o bad cholesterol). Studies have revealed that persons who consumed 2 ounces (56 grams) of fenugreek seed each day had 14% lower cholesterol levels after 6 months. These persons had also reduced their risk for a heart attack by over 25%.

Atherosclerosis

Fenugreek is used for atherosclerosis (hardening of the arteries).

Skin lesion treatment

Fenugreek poultice is used to reduce the pain and inflammation in skin lesions like eczema, wounds, ulcers, burns, boils and cellulitis (infection of the tissue beneath the skin).

Mouth ulcer treatment

Fenugreek is used to treat mouth ulcers.

Chapped lip treatment

Fenugreek is used to treat chapped lips.

Baldness treatment

Fenugreek is used to treat baldness.

Heart burn and acid reflux treatment

Fenugreek is used to treat gastritis (inflammation of the stomach), heart burn and acid reflux since it contains mucilage which coats the stomach and intestines. The seeds can be sprinkled on the food to reap this benefit or a teaspoon can be swallowed with water before the meal.

Digestive aide

Fenugreek is used to improve the digestion. It is also used for upset stomachs.

Anorexia treatment

Fenugreek is used for anorexia or loss of appetite.

Constipation prevention

Fenugreek prevents constipation.

Antipyretic

Fenugreek is used to reduce fever. 1 teaspoon of fenugreek seeds can be consumed three times a day together with honey and lemon.

Breast enlargement

Fenugreek is used for breast enlargement since it promotes the growth of new breast cells and increases the size and fullness of the breasts. Some herbalists recommend taking 3 grams of fenugreek each day for this purpose.

Breast milk production

Fenugreek seeds and leaves can improve the amount of breast milk produced by breastfeeding women. Studies have shown that it can cause an increase of over 500% within 24 to 72 hours. Some herbalists recommend taking 500 mg of powdered fenugreek seed three times a day for this purpose.

Aphrodisiac

Fenugreek is used to boost the libido and for erectile dysfunction.

Ease menopausal symptoms

Fenugreek is used to ease the symptoms of menopause like hot flashes and mood fluctuations due to its estrogen-like properties.

Ease PMS symptoms

Fenugreek is used to ease the symptoms of PMS due to its estrogen-like properties. It is also used to reduce menstrual pain.

Labor induction

Fenugreek is used to induce labor since it stimulates uterine contractions. When taken just before deliver it can cause the baby to have an unusual odor which can be confused with maple syrup urine disease.

Muscle pain treatment

Fenugreek poultice is used to treat muscle pain.

Arthritis treatment

Fenugreek is used to treat arthritis. The poultice is used to reduce the pain and inflammation of gout.

Weight loss

Some studies show that fenugreek seed extract can lower daily fat intake in men who are overweight.

Improve exercise performance

Fenugreek is used to improve exercise performance. A study showed that taking 500 mg of fenugreek extract for 2 months increased testosterone levels and decreased body fat.

Asthma treatment

Fenugreek is used to treat asthma and bronchitis. It is also used for chronic coughs and tuberculosis.

Sore throat treatment

Fenugreek is used to treat sore throats.

Kidney disorders

Fenugreek is used for kidney disorders. It is thought to reduce the amount of calcium oxalate in the kidneys which contributes to the formation of kidney stones.

Beriberi treatment

Fenugreek is used to treat beriberi which is caused by vitamin B1 (thiamine) deficiency.

Detoxification

Fenugreek is used for detoxification.

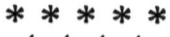

* * * * *

3

SAFETY PRECAUTIONS

1. Pregnant women should not use fenugreek since it can stimulate uterine contraction.

2. Some children have been reported to have become unconscious after drinking fenugreek tea.

3. Persons taking anti-diabetes medications should avoid fenugreek since it can also lower blood sugar levels.

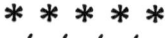

4

DRUG INTERACTIONS

1. Fenugreek can interact with antidiabetes medications and lower blood sugar levels.

2. Fenugreek can slow blood clotting and cause bleeding in persons taking anticoagulant and antiplatelet medications. Examples of these medications include aspirin, clopidogrel (Plavix), dalteparin (Fragmin), enoxaparin (Lovenox), heparin and warfarin (Coumadin).

* * * * *

5

HERBAL RECIPES

Fenugreek Poultice

Equipment

Cheesecloth or old cotton sheet strips

***

Ingredients

1 tablespoon powdered fenugreek

Boiling water

***

Instructions

1. Add enough boiling water to the fenugreek to wet it and make a thick paste.

2. Spoon the fenugreek paste onto the cheesecloth (or bed sheet strips) to make the poultice.

3. To use, apply the poultice to the affected area and cover with another piece of hot, wet cloth. Replace the hot, wet cloth when it cools with another hot one to keep the poultice hot.

*****

Fenugreek Tea

Equipment
Tea pot or kettle

***

Ingredients
1 teaspoon of finely crushed fenugreek

1 cup of boiling water

Honey to taste (optional)

***

Instructions
1. Put the fenugreek in a tea pot or kettle, add the boiling water and let it steep while covered for 10 -15 minutes.

2. Add honey (if using) to suit your taste before drinking.

*****

Fenugreek Infusion

Equipment

Glass jar with tight fitting lid

***

Ingredients

1 teaspoon fenugreek

1 cup boiling water

***

Instructions

1. Place the fenugreek in the glass jar and add the boiling water to fill the jar.

2. Close the lid and let the mixture steep for 4 hours to 14 hours (overnight).

3. Strain the fenugreek and the infusion is ready for consumption.

4. Store the infusion in the refrigerator to lengthen its life.

***

Tips

1. This infusion can be used to make sauces and incorporate the healing benefits of fenugreek in your diet.

*****

Fenugreek Syrup

Equipment

Saucepan

Jar with airtight lid

***

Ingredients

1 quart (1000 ml) filtered water

1 cup fenugreek

1 cup honey

***

Instructions

1. Place the water and fenugreek in a saucepan and bring to a boil.

2. Reduce the heat and let it simmer while it is partially covered until the volume is reduced to half the original volume.

3. Strain the mixture through a sieve or cheesecloth to remove the fenugreek.

4. Measure 1 pint (500 ml) of the liquid and add the honey.

5. Cook for a few minutes as you stir it so that it thickens.

6. Store the syrup in an airtight container in the fridge for up to 2 months.

***

Tips

1. This syrup can be used for coughs.

FENUGREEK

*****

Fenugreek Tincture

Equipment

Glass jar with tight fitting lid

Dark tincture bottles

Cheesecloth

Labels

*

Ingredients

7 oz (200 gm) fenugreek

30 oz (1 liter) of 80-100 proof vodka

*

Instructions

1. Fill 1/3 of the glass jar with the fenugreek.

2. Add the vodka to completely fill the jar to the top.

3. Seal the jar and label it and store it in a dark place for 6 weeks ensuring that you shake them weekly.

5. After 6 weeks strain out the fenugreek with a cheesecloth and pour the tincture into dark tincture bottles.

6. Label the tincture bottles with the date and name of fenugreek used.

7. Store your herbal tinctures away from light and heat.

**

Fenugreek Infused Oil

Equipment

Double boiler

Large glass bowl

Sieve and cheesecloth

Sterilized dark jars

***

Ingredients

16 fl oz. (500 ml) vegetable oil like olive or sweet almond oil

8 oz. (250 grams) slightly crushed fenugreek

***

Instructions

1. Place the fenugreek and oil in the glass bowl ensuring that the oil covers the fenugreek. Simmer them in a double boiler for 1 hour at around 120 degrees Fahrenheit (49 degrees Celsius). Do not let the mixture boil. You can repeat this step several times after letting the oils cool to create more concentrated herb infused oils.

2. Strain the mixture through a sieve and cheesecloth into a clean jar and squeeze out as much oil as you can from the cheesecloth.

3. Label your jars and sStore your fenugreek infused oils in a cool dark place or in the refrigerator and use them within 3 months.

*****

Fenugreek Butter

Equipment

Large glass bowl

Electric mixer or stick blender or wire whisk

Molds such as ice cube trays (optional)

***

Ingredients

½ cup butter

2 tablespoons of finely crushed fenugreek

***

Instructions

1. Place the butter in a warm place so that it can soften.

2. Put butter and fenugreek in a large glass bowl and blend well until thoroughly mixed.

3. Refrigerate until it hardens. You can refrigerate it in molds or ice cube trays to give it a special shape.

###

ABOUT THE AUTHOR

Marian Kim is an experienced alternative medicine practitioner.

*****

OTHER BOOKS BY THE AUTHOR

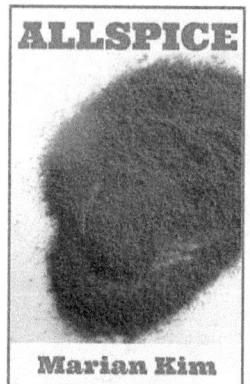

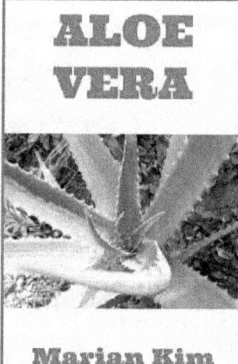

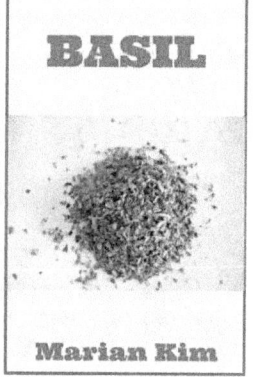

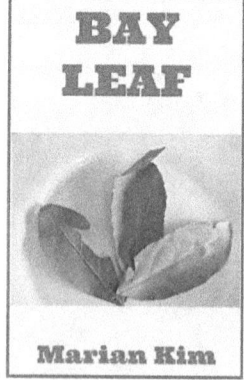

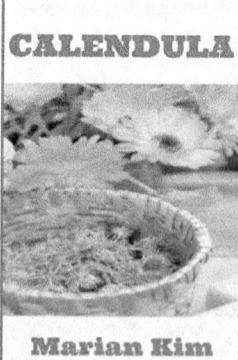

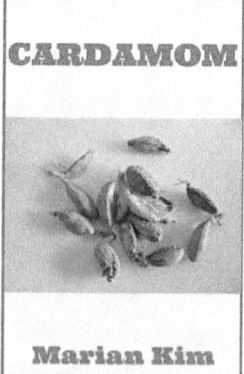

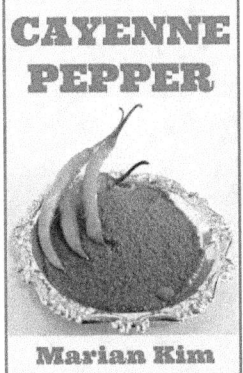

CAYENNE PEPPER

Marian Kim

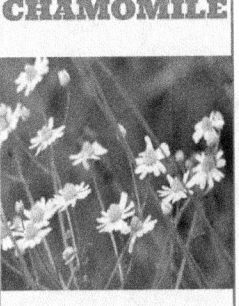

CHAMOMILE

Marian Kim

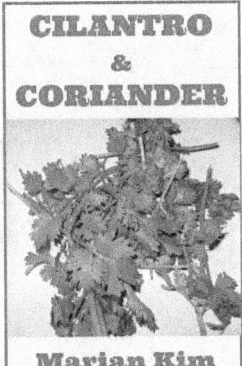

CILANTRO & CORIANDER

Marian Kim

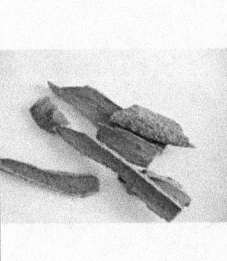

CINNAMON

Marian Kim

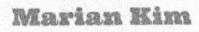

CLOVES

Marian Kim

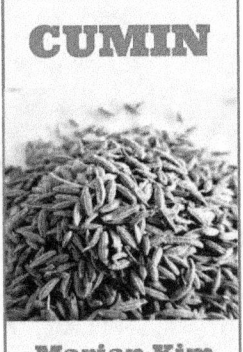

CUMIN

Marian Kim

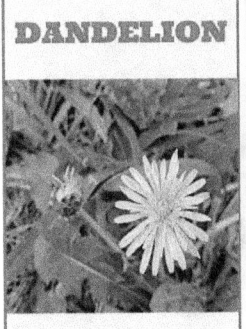

DANDELION

Marian Kim

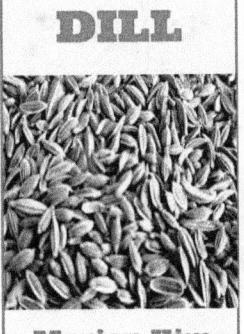

DILL

Marian Kim

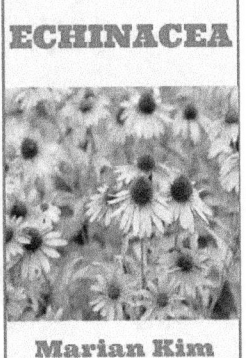

ECHINACEA

Marian Kim

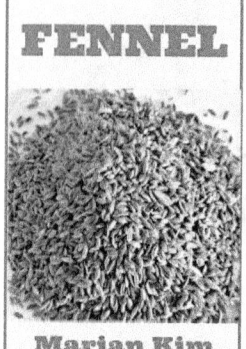

FENNEL

Marian Kim

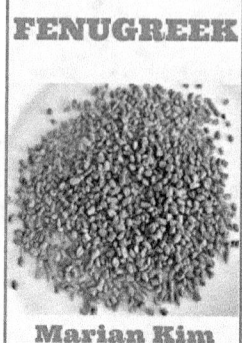

FENUGREEK

Marian Kim

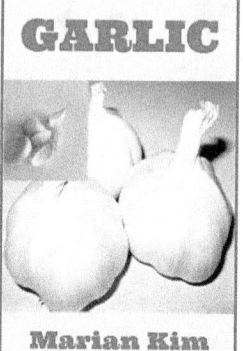

GARLIC

Marian Kim

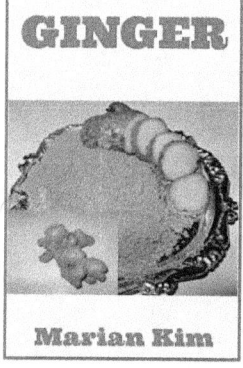

GINGER

Marian Kim

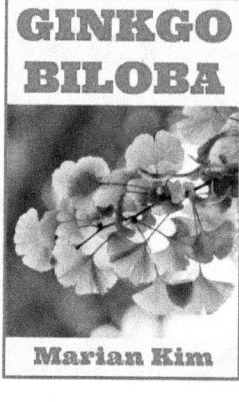

GINKGO BILOBA

Marian Kim

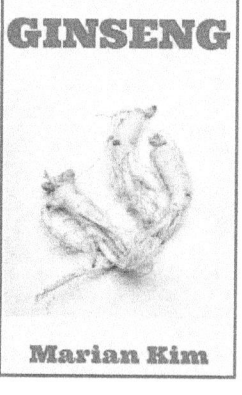

GINSENG

Marian Kim

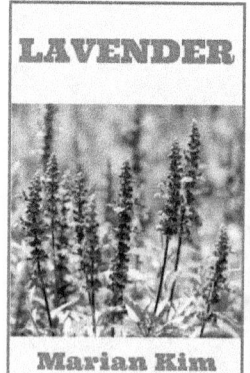

LAVENDER

Marian Kim

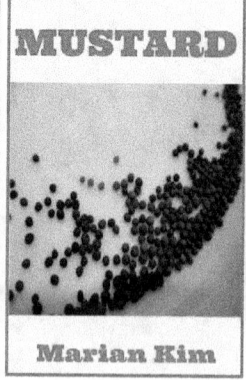

MUSTARD

Marian Kim

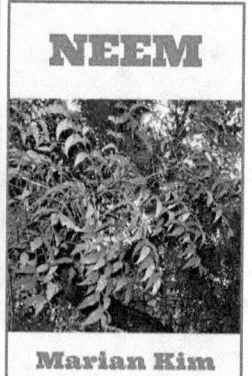

NEEM

Marian Kim

NUTMEG & MACE

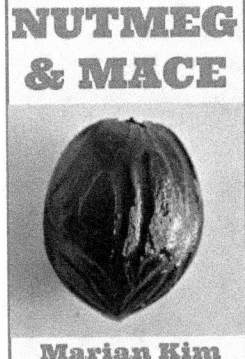

Marian Kim

OREGANO

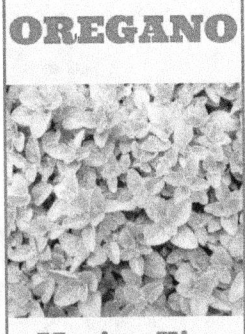

Marian Kim

PAPRIKA

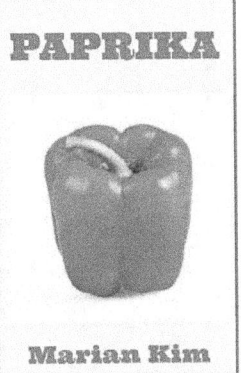

Marian Kim

PARSLEY

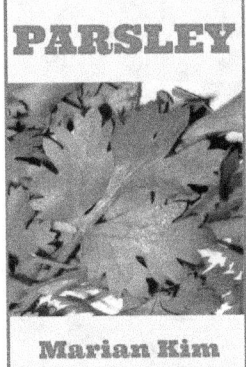

Marian Kim

BLACK & WHITE PEPPER

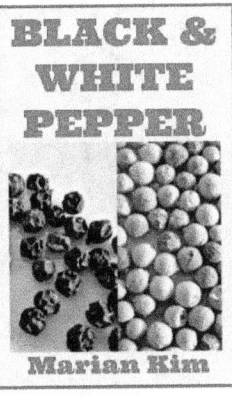

Marian Kim

PEPPERMINT

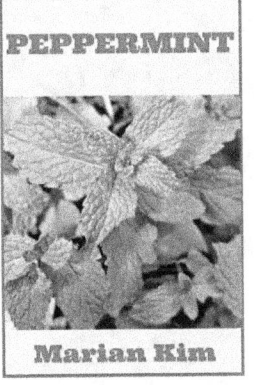

Marian Kim

ROSE HIPS

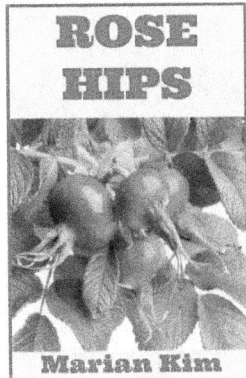

Marian Kim

ROSE PETALS

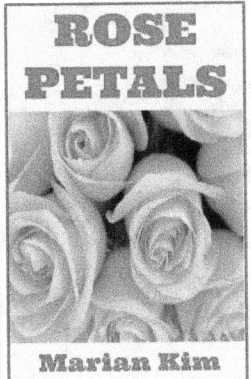

Marian Kim

ROSEMARY

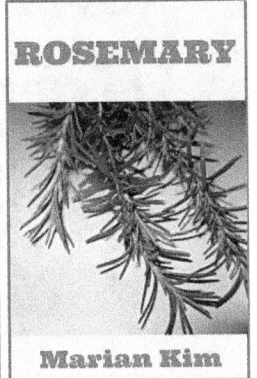

Marian Kim

SAGE

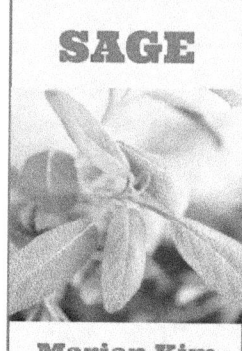

Marian Kim

ST. JOHN'S WORT

Marian Kim

STAR ANISE

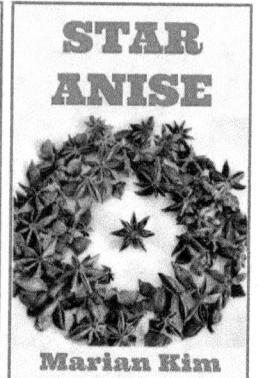

Marian Kim

STINGING NETTLE

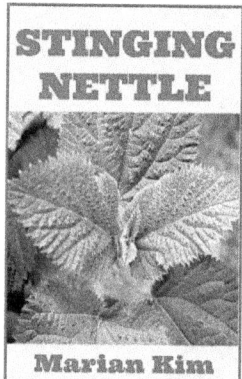

Marian Kim

THYME

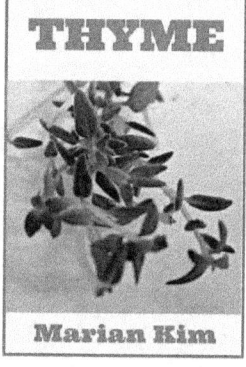

Marian Kim

TURMERIC

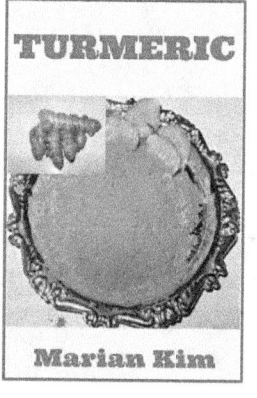

Marian Kim

WITCH HAZEL

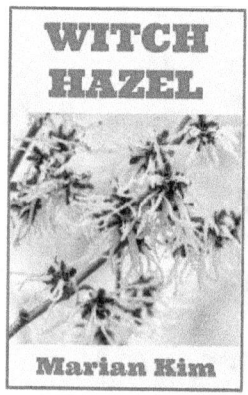

Marian Kim

YARROW

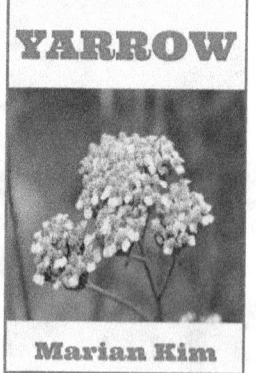

Marian Kim

*****